CONTENTS

INTRODUCTION

"You should eat healthy."

"Health is wealth."

"Healthy eating is the key to long life."

You might have come across these words and even uttered them at one point or the other. Healthy living is a quest that many people are striving to achieve. Healthy living begins with our food choices. This is still a challenge to many.

To eat well, you must know what to eat, how much to eat and what not to eat. Most people have a rough idea of what it means to eat clean and healthy. You should avoid processed sugars, trans fats, and junk food. Healthy dieters know that it goes deeper than this though. Some foods presumed healthy have countless negative health effects. Others, known as fad diets, are harmful, yet so many people keep falling for them.

So, how can you begin healthy eating?

Welcome to the plant-based diet.

The plant-based diet is pretty much what it sounds like. What you eat comes from plants. So fruits, nuts, seeds, legumes, and whole-grains are all part of the diet. As you can already tell, a plant-based diet is more or less a vegetarian/vegan diet.

This diet involves many health benefits.

For example, it helps in disease prevention and also supports **weight loss**. Also, it improves **fertility, cognitive function, metabolism, and digestive health**. It also combats so-called lifestyle diseases. The best part is that so many foods fall in the plant-based category, meaning the diet is sustainable. A plant-based diet will provide you with enough nutritious food as a vegan or vegetarian.

As with any other diet, a transition may not be as easy and straightforward as it seems. Many challenges may arise, ranging from:

- What to eat
- How to balance your meal to prevent having a deficiency of some nutrients
- Knowledge of what is good and what is not
- Gaining confidence about the diet

Many myths surround the diet, and they need to be debunked for one to benefit.

This book will take you through the plant-based diet step by step. It will empower you through knowledge and direction. Scientific evidence and facts back the diet, and you will know exactly how the body changes.

When you finish reading, you'll have the know-how to transition to the plant-based diet. This book also has simple recipes that you can prepare now.

A plant-based diet is one step to achieving good health. **Let's begin the journey together!**

CHAPTER ONE: WHAT IS A "PLANT-BASED DIET"?

A PLANT-BASED DIET IS AN EATING PLAN OF FOODS DERIVED solely from plants. The diet is all about the following principles:

1. A plant-based diet includes vegetables, legumes, fruits, seeds, and nuts. These food groups should make up the majority of your meals.
2. Emphasis on whole foods, which means minimization of any processed food.
3. Animal products should ideally be limited or eliminated from the meal plan. This is wholly dependent on the approach that you choose. If you want your meals to be 100% plant-based, then you should not consume any animal products. If you choose to consume some products, you must ensure that you cut them as much as possible.
4. Elimination of most refined foods such as flour, processed oils, and added sugars.

5. You must pay special attention to the (Whole Food Plant-Based) WFPB guidelines. The rules propose the eating of food in its most natural form. Proponents of WFPB aim to buy fresh food always. For processed foods, select the ones with the least number of added ingredients.

If the plant-based diet sounds appealing, know the difference between vegetarian and vegan. This will help you plan your meals better.

Vegan vs. Vegetarian Diet

The terms vegan and vegetarian are used interchangeably by many people. Still, few can articulate the differences, as the two are quite similar.

You know how all thumbs are considered to be fingers while not all fingers are considered to be thumbs? This is the perfect analogy to depict the differences between a vegan and a vegetarian diet. All vegans are vegetarians but not all vegetarians are vegans.

Veganism and vegetarian food preferences are all part of the plant-based diet. They all lean toward consuming more plants and fewer (if any) animal/animal products.

Vegetarian diet

As, you know, a vegetarian consumes plant-based foods. This includes fresh vegetables, grains, nuts, seeds, and fruits.

Not all vegetarians are the same, though. Different degrees and categories of vegetarianism exist. All are dependent on their inclusion of eggs and dairy into their diet. The classifications are:

1. Lacto ovo vegetarians: This group consumes eggs and dairy products. The group only abstains from eating animal flesh.
2. Lacto vegetarians: This group consumes dairy but not eggs or any animal meat.
3. Ovo vegetarians: This group eats eggs but not dairy or any animal meat
4. Vegans: Vegans do not consume any animal meat or animal-derived products.
5. Fruitarian. This category consumes fruits only
6. Pescatarian. This group consumes fruits, vegetables, eggs, dairy, and seafood.
7. Raw vegan. This group only eats raw vegetables.

To itemize, vegetarians do not consume:

- Any animal meat such as pork, beef, fish, and game (meat from wild animals)
- Any poultry such as duck, turkey, and chicken
- Any insects
- Animal protein such as gelatin and rennet
- Any stocks or fats that are derived from slaughtered animals

That said, some vegetarians might consume the following by-products:

- Dairy products such as milk, yogurt, kombucha, and cheese
- Eggs from poultry
- Honey and honey products from bees

Vegan diet

The vegan diet is the strictest form of the vegetarian diet. Vegans have a very clear cut diet, which prohibits the consumption of any animal meat and their byproducts. Anything that comes from animals, including honey from bees, is forbidden.

Most vegans consider their food preference to be "a way of life'. They seek to exclude themselves from any form of animal cruelty or exploitation. Killing animals for food or derivatives such as leather is considered cruel. Eating their produce is deemed exploitation. Ergo, their core philosophy revolves around compassion toward and protection of animals.

Most vegans extend their beliefs beyond diet. They are against the use of animal derivations such as leather, wool, beeswax, and silk. So a strict vegan would not have leather seats in their car nor use a beeswax candle.

Reasons for Vegetarianism or Veganism

Now we can discuss why the differences between vegetarian and vegan exist in the first place. As discussed, the most prominent reason why most vegetarians opt for the diet is health. The vegetarian diet is very low in unhealthy fats, carbs, and saturated sugars. This makes it the best choice for anyone who wishes to lead a healthier lifestyle. Some people may have moral and political reasons. This is rarely the case if they do not opt for the entire vegan ideology.

Vegans are very strict and their practice is very straightforward. For the full vegan diet, health reasons are rarely the cause of their food choice. Most vegans are influenced by their moral, ethical, political, or religious beliefs. Many vegans are also highly concerned with the environmental impact of most processes. They aim to refrain from supporting anything that causes pollution.

Intersection of Vegetarianism, Veganism, and a Plant-Based Diet

The term "plant-based" has different meanings to different people. For some, it means scaling up the intake of vegetables and fruit. For others, it means entirely shifting to plant-based foods. Most people choose to shift entirely, which makes them vegetarians. If you are here, it is up to you to determine the type of vegetarian that you want to be. If you would like to consume plants only, you are by default a vegan.

A plant-based diet is one of the healthiest food choices that a person can ever make. To decide where to begin, there is a need to know the differences between whole and non-whole foods. With the knowledge, you can make better decisions about what to buy and what not to.

Whole vs Non-Whole Foods

Whole foods comprise any food that is in its natural form with little to no processing done. Whole foods are also devoid of any artificial additives. Any food that falls in this category is considered to be one of the healthiest options. The fact that they are not processed means that all nutrients are retained. Fruits, vegetables, nuts, and cereals fall in this category.

Non-whole foods comprise any foods that have undergone processing. Most processed foods are also laden with artificial additives, sugars, and preservatives. Most have one or many nutrients distorted during processing. For example, packaged wheat flour is a non-whole food. It has added sugars, preservatives, and minerals.

Most ingredients in a plant-based diet are whole. To make sure that you keep it this way, ensure that you buy fresh produce and fruits. Avoid their processed counterparts. You can be sure that canned corn is non-whole, regardless of the fact that the main ingredient is corn. Thus, the healthier alternative would be to buy corn on the cob.

Note when you consume plant-based food at night you get nutrients such as vitamin B6. They are just less nutritious and healthy compared to their counterparts. Why? As processing takes place, less-nutritious ingredients such as salt, sugar, and fats increase. Thus, beneficial mineral and vitamin content decrease.

Chapter Summary

- A plant-based diet focuses on whole vegetables, fruits, seeds, and nuts.
- You can either be a vegetarian or a vegan while on the plant-based diet.
- Some vegetarians tolerate animal products such as milk and poultry eggs. Vegans do not.
- A plant-based diet advocates for whole foods and reduction of non-whole foods.
- Whole foods comprise of any food in its natural, which has not been processed.
- Non-whole foods undergo some processing such as adding salt, flavors, or preservatives.

In the next chapter, you will learn about the benefits of the plant-based diet and why people switch to it.

CHAPTER TWO: BENEFITS AND WHY PEOPLE SWITCH

You are what you eat. To be healthy and fit, the food you eat matters.

As lifestyle disease becomes more common, we need a proper diet and nutrition. According to the CDC, malnutrition is the top contributor to preventable chronic diseases. Unhealthy food causes obesity, diabetes, some cancers, and heart diseases, and more. It is very sad to see people eat themselves to death.

A 2017 study featured in *The Lancet* revealed poor diet accounts for 1 in 5 adult deaths worldwide.

The WHO estimates that obesity has tripled over the last three decades. This has led to an increase in associated diseases. The two most prevalent are diabetes and heart ailments. Thirty-nine percent of adults are currently overweight globally, another staggering 17% are obese. In the United States, 69% of adults and 19% of children below 19 years are overweight. The WHO estimates that the numbers will keep increasing over time if people do not change.

Luckily, more people are realizing the negative effects of poor nutrition. A good number continues to adopt healthier diet options. The plant-based diet is one of the most preferred healthy diets. This is particularly among young people. A study from The Guardian showed a 350% increase in U.K. people opting for a plant-based diet since 2006. The majority of these people have adopted veganism.

The trend is very promising, and nutritionists want to promote the lifestyle globally.

Health Benefits of a Plant-Based Diet

Weight Loss

The science of weight loss is very simple. You need to use up more calories than you consume. Assuming you're consistent, shifting to a plant-based diet will help you lose weight. This is due to the following facts:

1. A plant-based diet has very high fiber content. Fiber is very filling. This means that you will end up eating less, and you will remain full for longer. As a result, the calorie intake will decrease. The body will then begin to burn up more body fat to compensate for the energy deficiency.
2. A plant-based diet contains complex carbohydrates. Complex carbs are usually absorbed much slower into the bloodstream compared to simple-carbs. As a

result, you are likely to be fuller for longer, preventing excess calorie consumption. Also, since glucose is absorbed slowly, it does not get stored as fat as often as a simple-carb meal would.

3. The diet is rich in minerals and nutrients. These nutrients help improve the diversity of gut bacteria. The diversity has a direct effect on weight loss in the following ways:

- Some gut bacteria produce chemicals that influence the production of hormones. When you eat, the body produces different hormones that affect your appetite. Some of these hormones include leptin, ghrelin, and peptide. The more and faster these hormones are produced, the faster and fuller you will feel. Ultimately, eating less will result in weight loss.
- When you eat high-fiber-content food, gut bacteria involved release short-chain fatty acids. These chemicals then trigger the release of appetite hormones, making you fuller faster.
- There are good gut bacteria and bad gut bacteria. Proper diet destroys bad gut bacteria and increases good bacteria. Some bad bacteria are known to cause inflammation. The inflammation causes a release of chemicals such as lipopolysaccharide (LPS). LPS is often associated with issues such as insulin resistance. This resistance results in weight gain. More good bacteria promotes weight loss.
- Gut bacteria affect nutrient absorption and the storage of energy in the body. When you have diversity, there is a lower disposition of fat in body

cells. Fewer bacteria results in a faster conversion of fat to glucose. This results in weight gain.

1. People on a plant-based diet eat fewer total calories than meat eaters. Daily caloric intake is the most important determinant of weight loss.

According to Healthline, overweight people have fewer gut bacteria compared to healthier people. Eating nutritious food helps to promote bacterial diversity.

With weight loss and weight management, the prevalence of lifestyle diseases decreases. Thus, you will be less susceptible to diabetes, cardiovascular diseases, and weight-related cancers.

Lower Prevalence of Blood Pressure

A plant-based diet is rich in potassium and vitamin B6. Both occur with stable blood pressure. Whole grains, vegetables and fruits, seeds, and nuts contain high potassium and B6.

Notably, animal meat has little to no potassium. Thus, people who consume too few plants experience high blood pressure and cholesterol.

Lower Cholesterol

Plants do not contain any cholesterol. No plant has any cholesterol content. Even saturated sources like cacao and coconut do not have cholesterol. Vegans realize this benefit more than other vegetarians considering the following facts:

1. One egg has twice the amount of cholesterol you would get in a fast-food hamburger. Thus, *lacto ovo* vegetarians still consume a lot of cholesterol through eggs.
2. Dairy products such as cheese, milk, whipped cream, and butter have cholesterol. Thus, most vegetarians who consume them are still exposed to cholesterol.

If you are a vegetarian, be wary of cholesterol in poultry eggs and dairy. It would be prudent to cut intake as much as possible.

Increased Energy

Plants contain many minerals and vitamins that are excellent for energy. When we feed our body with nutritious food, we stimulate the thyroid gland. This supports energy metabolism. The thyroid gland's function is to regulate the following body activities:

- Breathing
- Metabolism
- Bodyweight
- Body temperature
- Heart rate

Whenever you need more energy, the thyroid gland responds

by producing hormones T3 and T4. Both control energy production. Thus, a healthy thyroid gland will have you rejuvenated throughout the day.

Poor diet is known to result in conditions such as hyperthyroidism. The condition causes the release of an abnormally high amount of thyroid hormone. This results in rapid heartbeat, extreme fatigue, and general low energy. A study from nutritionists showed a 52% increase in normal thyroid function among plant-based dieters.

Note when you consume plant-based food at night you get nutrients such as vitamin B6. This vitamin is imperative for relaxation and rest. The result is a well-regulated nervous system. When you get proper rest at night, you are likely to feel much more energetic the following day.

For better thyroid function, eat leafy vegetables. These are rich in magnesium, selenium, iodine, antioxidants, maca, and potassium.

Healthy Skin, Nails, and Hair

The skin is the largest organ in the body. It goes without saying that it should be one of the most protected organs in the human body. What we put into our bodies will always show on the outside. Some of the key reasons why a plant-based diet has a positive effect on the skin are:

1. The diet, particularly fruits and vegetables have very high water content. Greater intake means more hydrated skin, making it more supple and healthier.

2. A plant-based diet is **rich in antioxidants**. Antioxidants work by eliminating free radicals from the body, which then reduce inflammation. Most skin conditions such as acne and eczema are as a result of inflammation. A reduction of which results in a clearer and healthier skin.
3. Most nuts and seeds contain **Omega-3 fatty acids** which help to promote healthier cells. According to Dr. Andrew Stoll, a renowned author, every cell in the human body requires omega 3 to function. Omega 3 helps control inflammation and protects the cell membrane. Thus, the skin, as with all other organs, will be healthier.

Increased Cognitive Function

A plant-based diet helps reduce cognitive decline and impairment. As with lifestyle diseases, there has been a gradual increment of cognitive ailments. These include Alzheimer's and dementia over the years. The CDC estimates that the number will triple over the next few decades.

Currently, mental health disorder plague over 5 million Americans. Experts assert that diet, drugs, and alcohol are to blame. Unhealthy diets cause inflammation of the cell membranes in the brain. This results in advancement of the diseases. A plant-based diet helps reduce neurological ailments in the following ways:

1. Reduced neurological inflammation: Free radicals,

which only antioxidants can negate, can cause inflammation. Free radicals are very destructive, causing severe inflammation to the brain membrane. The result is neurological ailments and disorders such as:

- Alzheimer's
- Parkinson's
- Dementia
- ADHD
- Depression and anxiety

A diet rich in antioxidants results in the effective neutralization of free radicals. With reduced inflammation, you are likely to feel sharper and chances of developing neurological conditions are very slim.

1. **Mitochondrial biogenesis**: Mitochondria are cell organelles that are responsible for energy production. The production of energy takes place through a process known as oxidative phosphorylation. This occurs when oxygen and nutrients combine. In some instances, defective mitochondria inhibit ability to produce ATP. In such a case, free radicals in the body increase, producing neurodegenerative diseases.

A plant-based diet facilitates mitochondrial biogenesis, the creation of healthy mitochondria. With the increase in healthy mitochondria, there is lower production of free radicals.

1. **Omega- 3 benefits**: The brain is made up of millions of cells that have very specific building blocks. Fatty acids are amongst the key building blocks found in Omega 3. Fatty acids help improve brain function by increasing fluidity in the cell membranes. The fluidity helps in memory development and retention. That's imperative for learning and prevention of ailments such as dementia.
2. Most importantly, fats help in the development of the **brain's growth hormone** known as **BDNF**. This hormone helps promote cell regeneration in the brain, making it healthier. Your predisposition toward ADHD, depression, and bipolar disorders will decrease.

Celebrities Who Have Adopted a Plant-Based Diet

Unsurprisingly, many celebrities embrace the diet. Some of the top plant-based dieters include:

Ariana Grande

Ariana Grande is an award-winning musician, songwriter, and actress. The superstar went vegan in 2014 and has never looked back. Grande credits her vivacious energy, lean body, stamina, and glowing skin to the diet.

In an interview with Mirror, Grande said her decision to go

vegan came from her love of animals. Grande believes killing animals for meat is cruel, so she won't support the practice. Also, she believes a plant-based diet will lead to a longer, happier life.

In a follow-up interview with *V* magazine, Grande said she did not think it prudent for humans to drink cow's milk. As a pure vegan, Grande admits that it is very difficult for her to eat out. Thus, most of the time she just has to go home and prepare her meals herself.

Miley Cyrus

Miley Cyrus is also an award-winning singer, actress, songwriter, and philanthropist. Gluten and lactose intolerance prompted her to go vegan in 2012. The diet change worked wonders for her, and Cyrus credits her weight loss and health to the diet.

Cyrus is currently one of the most vocal vegan celebrities. She champions the lifestyle change via social media. In one post, Cyrus wrote that the diet had protected her from preventable diseases over the years.

Cyrus's diet change has affected all areas of her life. In an interview, she explained that her vegan lifestyle goes deeper than just what she eats. Cyrus does not wear any clothes made from animals such as fur and leather. She commissions custom pieces from designers like Louis Vuitton made from eco-friendly materials. Through her lifestyle, Cyrus hopes she can promote "cruelty-free fashion".

Peter Dinklage

Peter Dinklage is an American actor famed as Tyrion Lannister on Game of Thrones. The Grammy-award winning actor has been a vegetarian since childhood. In scenes where Dinklage can be seen eating "meat", he recently disclosed that it was tofu or fake meat.

Just like most vegetarians, Peter Dinklage is a huge animal protection activist. Dinklage has worked with PETA before to oppose abandonment of huskies.

Tennessee Titans

The Tennessee Titans are some of the greatest athletes of all time. An accident prompted many of them to go vegan. It all began when the wife to one of the players, Derrick Morgan, began making vegan meals for her husband. Charity Morgan, the wife, is a chef and always prepared meals for her husband to carry to practice. Derrick noticed an increase in energy and reduced inflammation on the new diet. As such, he soon gave up meat for athletic performance. The other athletes began stealing his food, remarking how delicious it was. Like Derrick, they felt more energetic afterward. Soon, Derrick's wife was preparing meals for 12 athletes. Most of the athletes turned vegan.

Charity also transitioned to the diet and introduced it to their children. Amazed by the health outcomes, Charity turned full-time vegan chef. There are so many food options, and the now renowned chef says that her clients have never had the same meal twice. She calls her foods "healing".

Cost Benefits of a Plant-Based Diet

A plant-based diet is very cost-efficient. Proponents assert that the diet has helped them save costs in many ways, some of which include:

Reduced Healthcare Costs

Health problems can create a financial burden due to increased medical treatment costs. Some people even end up going bankrupt after treatment. Some medical conditions cannot be reversed, leading to ongoing medication usage. For example, diabetics need daily insulin shots to stabilize their blood glucose.

Reduced Food Costs

On average, a plant-based diet is cheaper than any other diet. The ingredients that make up a plant-based diet cost less than meat products. In addition, the variety of food choices in a plant-based diet can be more filling. You'll eat less and spend less on food.

According to Thinkmoney, an animal-based diet is expensive worldwide. A recent study published in the Journal of Hunger & Environmental Nutrition has found that people who adopt a vegetarian diet save an average of $750 each year on groceries compared to people who eat meat. In the study, researchers put together two seven-day meal plans, one including meat and one excluding. They found that the items on the meat plan were, on average, more expensive. This lays to rest the myth that healthy diets cost more.

Chapter Summary

A plant-based diet is the healthiest choice that any person can make including the following benefits:

- Weight loss
- Normal blood pressure
- Low cholesterol
- Increased energy

For some of those reasons, many celebrities have turned to the plant-based diet.

In the next chapter, we will demystify assumptions surrounding the plant-based diet.

CHAPTER THREE: 10 COMMON MYTHS OF A PLANT-BASED DIET

If you are considering going for a plant-based diet, here is a list of common myths you should be aware of. Not all information out there is factual in our internet-browsing and opinion-based society. Thus, we must separate truth and myth to follow the diet.

Some of the most common myths include:

Myth #1: A Plant-Based Diet is Expensive

This is one of the most common myths that continue to negatively impact people who want to try out the diet. A plant-based diet isn't a fad diet where people spend hundreds to get "healthy". Everything plant-based is natural. A meal will likely cost you less than processed food, as we discussed in the previous chapter.

Furthermore, the fact that a plant-based diet is rich in fiber means that you will feel fuller for longer. This translates to less eating, hence lower costs. When you eat, say, bread and tea in the morning, you might feel like snacking after a few hours. The drastic rise and fall in sugar levels leave you hungry, and you must eat. A plant-based diet leaves you fuller, and which means more time between meals.

While we're talking expenses, let's consider the long term effects diets have. A plant-based diet decreases likelihood of expensive lifestyle diseases. You are better off preventing them from developing in the first place.

Myth #2: A Plant-Based Diet Does Not Have Enough Protein

This is a common myth that stems from the belief that animal meat is the only source of protein. Most people feel abstaining from animal meat will result in protein deficiency.

Meat is really not the only source. The truth is almost all sugar-free foods contain some level of protein in them. The recommended daily allowance (RDA) for protein is around 0.8grams/kg of body weight. That's quite achievable for people on a plant-based diet.

Some of the rich sources of protein include:

- Lentils
- Beans
- Most nuts
- Tofu
- Whole grains

- Seeds

Anyone can get enough protein from these foods, even gym rats. Be intentional in eating the outlined foods in large amounts.

Myth #3: A Plant-Based Diets Have No Variety

When most people think about a plant-based diet, a fear they have is that they won't be able to enjoy the same foods. Most people believe that a plant-based diet is very restrictive.

In truth, you can choose from a large variety of foods on a plant-based diet. Almost every food has an alternative that is just as tasty. The only difference is one of health. Almost all plant-based options are healthier. For example:

- Cooking with olive oil gives the food the same taste as cooking with other types of oils.
- Blends of nuts and spices can create cheese alternatives.
- You can sweeten desserts with fruits rather than processed sugars.
- You will not need soda because there are lots of fruit drinks.
- You can make snack bars using nuts as opposed to sugary snack bars.

There are so many plant-based recipes, and you can cook any food using a healthier alternative. Recreate your favorite meals using the plant-based alternative. You won't miss your meat-based foods.

Myth #4: You Will Lose Muscle on the Diet

This logic follows the protein-deficiency argument. People looking to grow their muscles may fret since they need a lot of protein to do so. Thus, they may be a bit reluctant to give up on chicken and other animal meats.

It's a myth.

According to the American Journal of Clinical Nutrition, protein source does not matter. So long as you consume as much as you need, it does not matter if the source is from nuts, legumes, or wherever you get it from.

So, rather than eat tons of meat, you eat tons of protein-rich plants and nuts. Also note weight training is as important as eating protein. Hit the gym and follow the workout with the relevant leafy greens, seeds, and beans.

Myth #5: A Plant-Based Diet Is Insufficient for Nutritional Needs

Some people think a plant-based diet lacks important nutrients, so you need supplements. This is not true. A plant-based diet is key to achieving optimal health. Dieters have access to almost all the nutrients they need. The one exception is vitamin B12, discussed later in this chapter.

Most plants have different nutrients and having variety in

your diet means you will get all you need. While taking supplements is not bad, it's unnecessary.

Myth #6: A Plant-Based Diet Is Not Safe for Pregnant Women

Pregnancy is a very tricky period for every woman, and doctors tell expectant mothers to eat well. If you're not on a plant-based diet already, pregnancy might be the wrong time to experiment. That said, you can attempt to include more plants in your diet.

For vegans, a plant-based diet will have no harm during pregnancy. In fact, it helps many since they're unlikely to gain excessive weight. Thus, the woman is less likely to suffer from gestational diabetes or high blood pressure.

A plant-based diet is fine for pregnant women. It's just not the best time to transition for women not already on the diet. All they have to do is increase their intake of nuts, dried fruit, soybeans, and nut butter. Also, many vegetables are very rich in folate and iron. The two are critical nutrients required by pregnant women.

Myth #7: You Will Always Be Hungry

Some people assume that you will always be hungry on a plant-based diet. Since you'll only eat plant-based foods, people think you'll be hungry. Actually, that couldn't be further from the truth. You will likely be fuller while on a plant-based diet due to the following reasons.

A plant-based diet is very rich in fiber. Thus, you will feel fuller faster and for longer.

A plant-based diet has complex carbs as opposed to the simple carbs that most regular diets have. Getting rid of spikes in blood glucose helps you to control any cravings you may have. This helps to control hunger.

Myth #8: You Will Have Less Energy

The assumption that you will have less energy on a plant-based diet is untrue. But, people who start the diet affirm that they feel more energetic than before.

A plant-based diet is very rich in iron, which is imperative for energy. Some nutrient-rich foods are spinach, chickpeas, cashews, beans, lentils, and kale. You can absorb even more iron if you eat such foods rich in vitamin C (tomatoes, oranges, broccoli). This translates to more energy.

Myth #9: Your Meals Will be Boring

As we have already stated, there are many recipes that you can adopt when you are on a plant-based diet. Thus, your meals will never have to be boring.

A plant-based diet does not change any meal set-up. You can still have a five-course meal, all plant-based. Most of the recipes have solid plant-based substitutes. That means you'll have interesting meals that mirror your favorites.

If your taste is posh, consider vegetarian cooking classes or online guides. In any case, this book will provide you with sample recipes that are wholesome and fun.

Myth #10: You Have to Go All-In

Shifting from one diet to another takes time. Thus, it would be erroneous to think that you have to shift automatically for it to work.

Trimming your meat intake lowers the risk of heart ailments, diabetes, and cancer. In other words, take your time to reduce meat intake. Slowly increase plant intake. Before long, your health will improve.

A plant-based diet does not have to be all-or-nothing. Listen to your body as you make the gradual change.

B12 Deficiency

Vitamin B12 is also known as cobalamin. It is one of the most important nutrients to the body. Usually, it's bad absorption that causes deficiencies. Unfortunately, vegans are likely to develop it.

Vitamin B12 is usually involved in vital body processes. Methyl transfer, myelin synthesis, nucleic acid metabolism, and body repair, for instance. All are necessary for red blood cells and normal neural functions.

Sadly, animal products are the major source of B12 leaving plant-based dieters vulnerable. Beef, pork, dairy products, and poultry eggs contain B12.

Once you transition to a plant-based diet, you'll need to keep this deficiency in mind. Some of the signs that you have a deficiency include:

Jaundiced/Pale Skin

People with vitamin B12 deficiency have a slight yellow tinge or paleness of the skin. That's jaundice. It usually occurs when red blood cell production slows.

Vitamin B12 plays a pivotal role in the production of the DNA required to make red blood cells. A deficiency, then, causes incomplete instructions, and the blood cells can't divide. The result is very few blood cells circulating the body. This is the reason why skin discoloration occurs.

Weakness and Fatigue

Red blood cells are responsible for the transport of oxygen throughout the body. When the body has too few of the cells, it means there is not enough oxygen moving throughout the body.

Normally, oxygen combines with the food consumed to produce ATP, which is energy. The lower the amounts of ATP produced, the lower the energy you are likely to give. Thus, you will witness more fatigue and weakness.

Sensations of Pins and Needles

This is the most telling sign that you have a vitamin B12 deficiency. It is also one of the most long-term signs associated with nerve damage. This presents as a tingling sensation. You will feel as if a million tiny needles are stabbing your fingers.

The nerve damage usually presents itself over time, and it is because of a lack of myelin. Usually, myelin surrounds the nerves to protect and insulate. With low B12, myelin production suffers and the nervous system cannot function properly.

The poor insulation of the nerves then causes increased sensitivity. This presents as the pricking sensation felt therein.

Mobility Changes

Any damage to the nerve endings is very retrospective in the long run. If left untreated, the damage can be so severe to the extent that it changes the way you move and walk. People with long-time B12 deficiency report poorer balance and coordination. This makes them more prone to issues such as falling.

Mobility changes may be one of the last symptoms that a person is likely to witness. Don't let it get to this point. You'll risk serious harm. If it does, seek immediate medical attention.

Breathlessness and Dizziness

B12 deficiency may leave you feeling a little anemic. The

result is shortness of breath and dizziness. Note that anemia is very serious, and you should never ignore such signs. Medical attention is of the utmost necessity at this point.

Blurred Vision

Blurred vision is also as a result of damage to the nervous system. Note that the damage to the nerves is not limited, and it affects almost all parts of the body.

Sensitive nerves such as the optic nerve that leads to your eyes are very damaging. The damage can cause disrupted nervous signals that travel from the eyes to the brain. In the end, you will experience disrupted vision, also known as optic neuropathy.

Extreme Mood Changes

Scientists have linked low B12 to mood and brain disorders such as dementia and depression. Experts suggest B12 deficiency leads to "the homocysteine hypothesis of depression".

The theory is that high homocysteine, caused by low B12, could interrupt signals to and from the brain. This causes mood changes. Low energy levels also feed into declining brain function. Then there's further aggravation of underlying conditions.

If you start experiencing mood swings out of the blue, you may want to take vitamin B12 supplements. Still, such conditions have many more causes. Not every neurological condition happens because of B12 deficiency.

A plant-based diet and Vitamin B12

Unfortunately, plants do not make vitamin B12. The only foods that contain the compound are meat, eggs, and poultry. Thus, there is no way for strict vegans to get the vital nutrients from any food consumed.

You must bear in mind when you transition to this diet that you have few B12 sources. This is most true for vegans. Thus, you need to supplement your diet with high dosage vitamin B12 pills. You can either decide to go for daily pills, which you have to take every day or weekly shots at your local hospital. Most people prefer taking pills, buyable over the counter at any pharmacy.

Protein Imbalance and How to Combat It

Protein imbalance occurs when you're unable to meet the body's protein requirements. Just like vitamins and other nutrients, protein is crucial. You must ensure you have enough.

As you know, proteins play a pivotal role in your muscles, skin, hormones, and enzymes. Basically, the compound is needed in all your body tissues. As we grow and develop, protein is of the utmost importance.

Most food has protein. Still, there is a chance that some

people, vegans especially, may be prone to some levels of deficiency. As we all know, animal meat and dairy are the richest sources of protein. Cutting them out from the diet means that you need to counter the imbalance. Most vegans have no problem achieving this since there are many plants rich in protein. Be that as it may, there are a few people who do.

When you begin a plant-based diet, you must pay attention to what you are eating. It is always good to be what I call an "intentional eater". So plan your meals. Track them. Be mindful. Finally, be attentive to the nutrients you're taking in.

In case you are not eating food rich in protein, the following signs may present.

Hair, Skin, and Nail Problems

Protein imbalance manifests itself in many ways, the most salient of which is in the hair, skin, and nails. The three are largely made of protein. A deficiency affects them directly. An imbalance can cause a drastic thinning of your hair, brittle nails, and rough skin. Note that these symptoms will only appear if your deficiency is relatively severe. Thus, witnessing them means that you have to seek medical attention fast.

Loss of Muscle Mass

Muscles are the largest reservoirs of protein. When you want to build muscles fast, you have to take a diet rich in protein and work out at the same time.

The body is self-sufficient. It will try to self-correct when there is some level of deficiency. When you take in too little protein, the body takes from skeletal muscles. It does so to keep more important tissues and muscles. The more the skeletal muscles taken away, the more you seemingly waste away.

Loss of muscle mass will be amongst the first signs of protein deficiency that you will realize. The condition is not permanent. Increase protein intake to reverse the problem.

Increased Severity of Infections

Protein deficiency takes a toll on the body's immune system. You will be more susceptible to infections, and their effect will be greater.

If you have an infection, you should be seeking medical help anyway. Still, if protein deficiency worsens the condition, you definitely need to seek medical attention.

How to Determine Your Protein Needs

Protein needs vary among different people. Many things determine how much protein that people need:

- Muscle mass
- Physical activity
- Age
- Bodyweight

Experts say that bodyweight determines protein needs. The recommended daily allowance (RDA) is usually 0.4 grams of protein for every pound. This equates to 0.8 grams per kg of a person's weight. For example, if you weigh 75kg (165 pounds), your daily protein intake should be 66 grams.

Note that this is the recommended minimum. You can consume as much protein as you wish, particularly when you are working out. When you are on a plant-based diet, some of the richest sources of protein include:

- Lentils
- Chickpeas
- Green peas
- Hempseed
- Tofu
- Seitan
- Asparagus
- Broccoli
- Mushrooms
- Brussels

Getting your daily recommended protein is so easy while on a plant-based diet. Aim to eat the above-mentioned food, and you will have no problems.

Chapter Summary

There are many unfounded myths that surround a plant-based diet. Some of the most common myths include:

1. A plant-based diet is expensive
2. The diet does not have enough protein
3. The diet is very restrictive
4. You will experience muscle loss on the diet
5. The diet has insufficient nutrients
6. The diet is not safe for pregnant women
7. You will always be hungry and have low energy
8. Your meals will be boring and you have to go all in

It is true that a plant-based diet is lacking in Vitamin B12, and you have to take supplements to combat it. Plus, if you have protein imbalance, you can combat any deficiencies. Your options are:

- Lentils
- Chickpeas
- Green peas
- Hempseed
- Tofu
- Seitan
- Asparagus
- Broccoli
- Mushrooms
- Brussels sprouts

In the next chapter, you will learn how to substitute meals in a meat-based diet.

CHAPTER FOUR: HOW TO SUBSTITUTE MEAT IN EVERYDAY MEALS

As you can see, eating a plant-based diet is nutritious, wholesome, and sustainable. If you're afraid to give up meat, though. Don't be. Most meat meals have plant-based substitutes. The fact is you will not have to say goodbye to any of your favorite meals.

Some of the best plant-based meat substitutes include:

Tofu

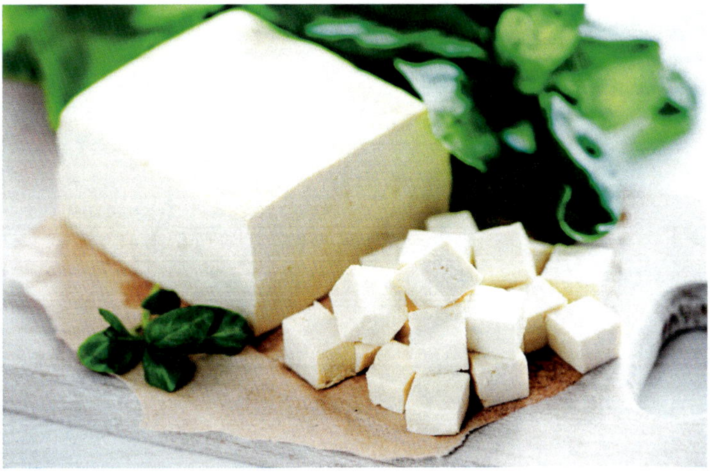

Tofu is a great substitute for most meat, including pork, chicken, and beef. You can also substitute it in seafood recipes, and it will be just as good. Tofu is popular among Asians, and it has been their staple food for ages. The plant tastes like meat, and all you have to do is replace any meat with it in your popular recipes. It's equally chewy and firm, making it suitable as an alternative. All you have to do is ensure that you freeze it before preparing meals.

Tempeh

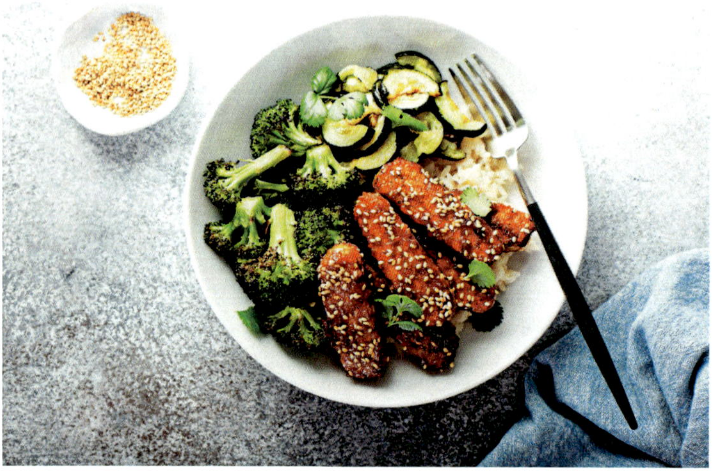

Tempeh has a more firm texture than tofu, the only other difference being that it is grainier. Since it is made from fermented soy sauce, you do not have to press it to make it firmer. All you have to do is slice it, grind it, and steam for a few minutes. The resultant emulates fish, so it's great for any recipe with fish as a key ingredient.

Seitan

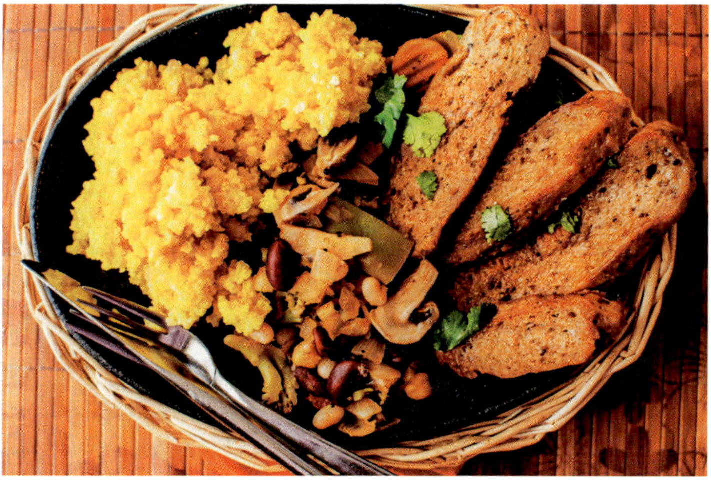

Seitan, just like tofu, has a meat-like texture and can be substituted in most meat recipes. The only difference between the two is that seitan has gluten. Hence it's unsuitable for people with gluten intolerance. If you have no such an intolerance, seitan works great to sub for meat, considering how sturdy it is.

Textured Vegetable Protein

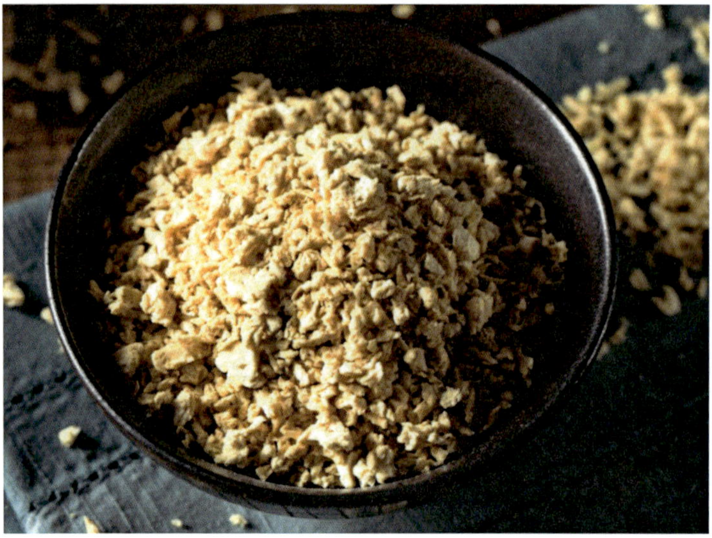

Textured vegetable protein (TVP) is a popular choice among vegans. This is particularly due to its inexpensive and easy-to-use characteristic. You can use TVP for just about anything. Since the ingredients come in granule form or chunks, it's flexible.

Jackfruit

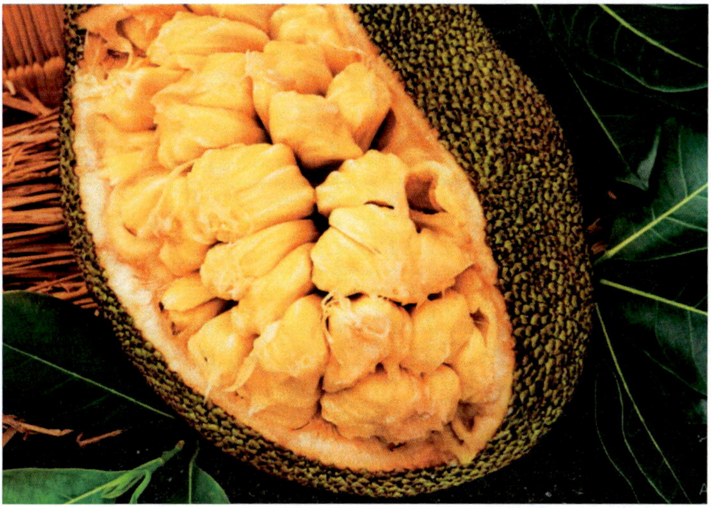

Jackfruit is a healthy tropical fruit that resembles meat in texture and taste. This ingredient makes a perfect stand-in for meat. All you have to do is cook it on a baking sheet for at least 15 minutes. The fruit is particularly perfect when making pork-based recipes.

Mushrooms

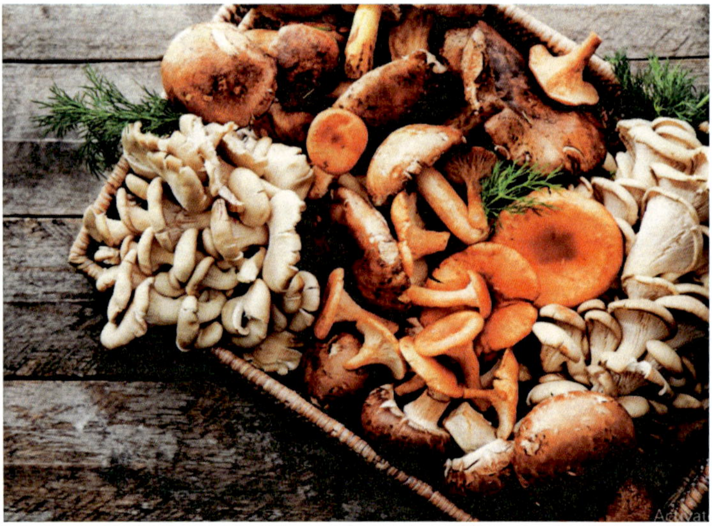

This is a favorite in most vegan households. Mushrooms can stand in for any meat. The color, texture, and flavor resemble meat, and you can use them in any meat recipe. The fact that they are healthier and more filling makes them great for weight loss meals.

Lentils

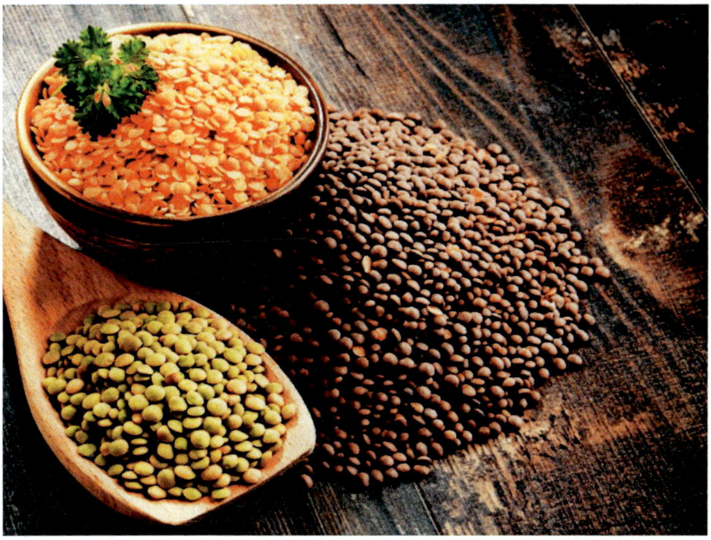

Lentils have been known to be a perfect stand-in for meat since time immemorial. This is particularly the case when you want to replace ground meat, without losing the taste. Lentils come in different colors and texture, and the major advantage is that they are cheap. Green lentils work great as minced meat in meatballs. Yellow lentils make great soups. Then there's red lentils, great in pies and tacos. Interchanging the lentils amongst the different recipes should be fun.

Eggplants

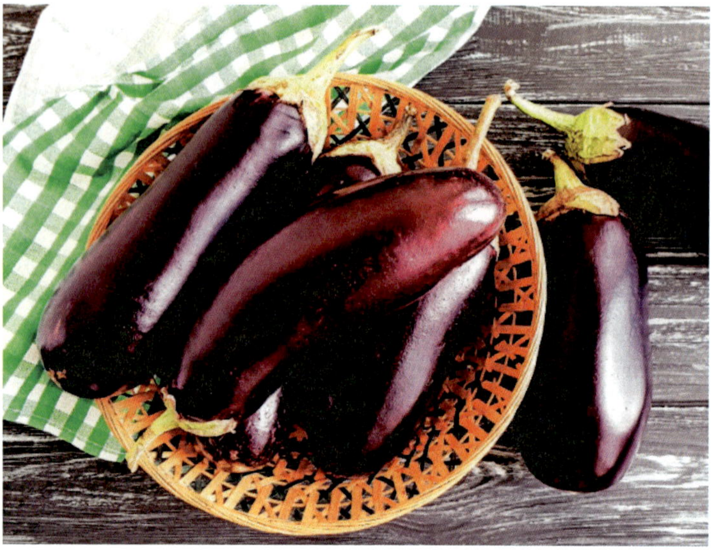

Eggplants are a perfect substitute for chicken. There is so much you can do with this ingredient. You can grill, bake and stuff, as you would a chicken. The meaty texture and savory flavor make it a killer poultry supplement. You will love it.

Commercial Plant-Based Options

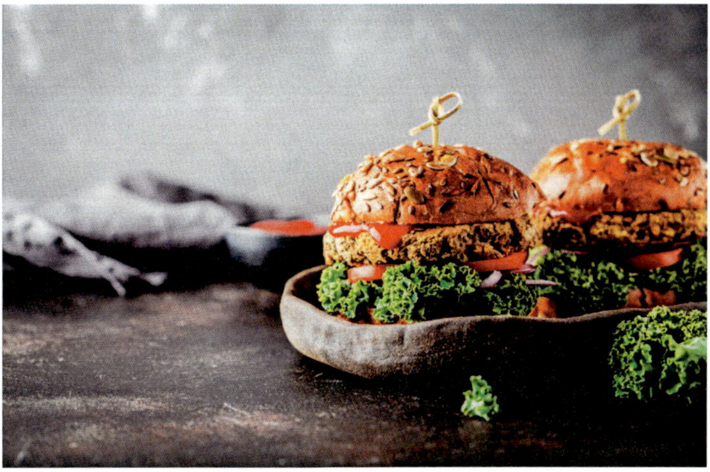

The increased demand for plant-based and vegan foods left a gap in the market. Companies needed to present more options to please vegetarians. Fortunately, vegans have not been left out anymore. There are many fast-food options that are designed solely for them, some of which include:

The Impossible Whopper from Burger King and Beyond Meat products. These are two of the most popular vegan fast foods, and they do not contain any animal products. The protein used is primarily from soy, potato, coconut oil, and hemp. Hemp accounts for the meat-like color.

Both burgers are fully vegan. People have affirmed that they are just as delicious as meat-based burgers. This just goes to show how unrestrictive a plant-based diet is. You can still enjoy any of your popular foods with no problems.

Making Plant-Based Choices When Going Out

Whenever you are going out, it is imperative that you become very intentional about the food that you eat. This ensures that you do not ruin your plant-based diet. Note that restaurants, like any other businesses, are most interested in profits. Thus, they may use some unscrupulous methods to deceive and try to get clients.

Home-cooked meals are the best for any vegetarian. Nonetheless, if you decide to go out, make sure the restaurant is credible. Some restaurants cater solely to vegetarians, and you are better off going to such places.

Most credible restaurants that offer a plant-based diet will tell you somehow. Restaurants often use three abbreviations to mark plant-based foods, V, VG, and VE. The three may either point out to vegetarian or vegan, and you should ask the waiters for help if you are not sure. Some restaurants use VO to denote "vegan option" and some use VA, or, "Vegan Available."

It also helps to ask the ingredients used in every meal. This is especially imperative for vegans, as some restaurants may use eggs in some of the recipes. The safest bet is to ask whenever unsure.

Chapter Summary

- There are so many vegetable supplements for meat recipes. Some of the most common supplements include tofu, jackfruit, tempeh, and more.

- Whenever you go out, ensure that you aim to eat a plant-based diet
- Some symbols for vegan food in restaurants include V, VE, VG, VA, and VO.

In the next chapter, you get simple vegetarian recipes that you can prepare anytime.

CHAPTER FIVE: PLANT-BASED RECIPES

Breakfast

Vegan Porridge

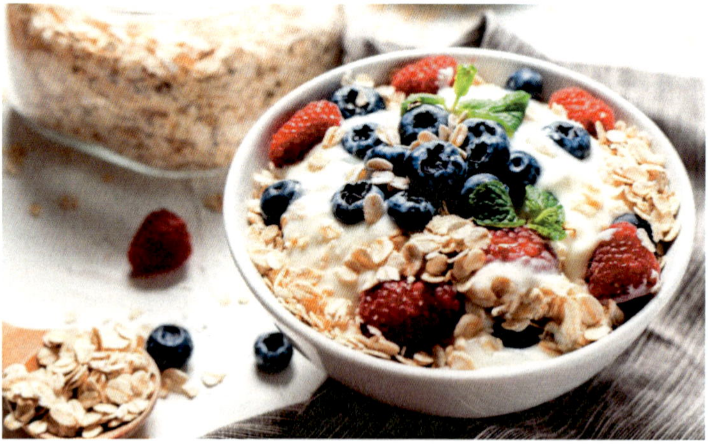

Serving size: 2

Estimated cooking time: 20 minutes

Ingredients

- 1 cup water/coconut milk
- 12 oz squash (butternut, kabocha, or acorn)
- 2 tbsp shredded coconut
- 3 tbsp sunflower seeds (lightly roasted). Can substitute with 2 tbsp coconut butter or coconut flakes
- Pure maple syrup/raw honey

Spices (Optional)

- ½ tbsp cinnamon
- 1 pinch turmeric powder
- 1 tbsp ginger powder
- Protein/collagen
- A pinch of salt

Toppings (all optional)

- Blueberries
- Blackberries
- Coconut cream
- Sesame seeds
- Tart cherries

Instructions

1. Chop the squash into large pieces and place them in a cooking pot. Add coconut oil and spices of your choice.
2. Sauté the squash for a few minutes and consistently turn them over every few minutes. To ensure that you are doing it right, check the top part. It should be well-coated with oil.
3. Add ½ cup of water into the pot and cover tightly with a lid. If you have a pressure cooker or an instant pot, it is much better since it cooks faster. Set a pressure cooker or instant pot to 5 minutes.
4. Remove squash from heat and blend using a hand blender or purée using a fork.
5. Once well blended, add all the other dry ingredients and milk. Stir thoroughly.
6. Return mixture to a pot and cook under medium heat. Your mixture should start bubbling after about two minutes, indicating it's ready.
7. Serve and add toppings of your choice.

Nutritional Value per Serving

Total calories: 331

Fiber: 8.7g

Plant protein: 7g

Saturated fat: 6.1g

Sodium: 180.4mg

Sugars: 16g

Carbohydrates: 43.1g

Fat: 17.7g

Banana-Nut Oatmeal

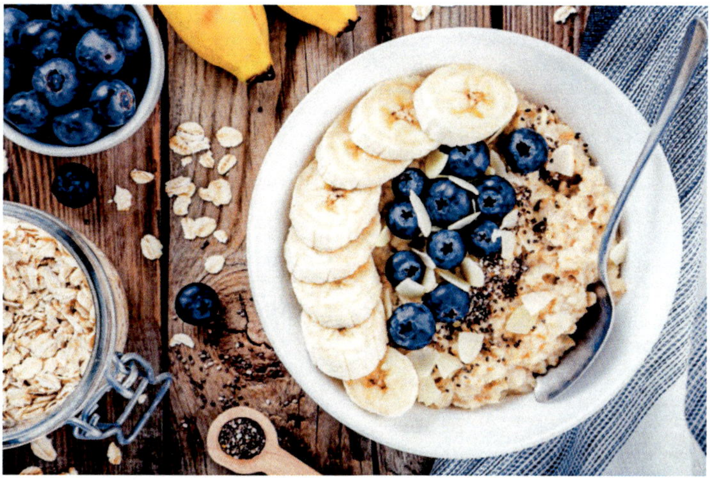

Serving size: 3

Estimated Time: 30 minutes

Ingredients

- 2 cups oats. There are many gluten-free options
- 2 medium bananas
- ½ cup almonds (sliced)
- 4 cups water
- 1 tablespoon cinnamon/vanilla

Instructions

1. Put water in a cooking pot and bring to boil over medium heat
2. In a small bowl, mix oats, one banana, and your preferred flavor.
3. Pour mixture into the boiling water, and stir slowly. Once it begins bubbling, lower the heat, and leave it for around 5-7 minutes.
4. At this point, the oatmeal should be thick enough. You can now add more almond/coconut milk, if it is too thick for you.
5. Serve in a small bowl. Cut the remaining banana into small pieces and add in the bowl. Also, add the almond pieces and any toppings of your choice.

Dried fruits are the perfect toppings, and you can add as many as you want.

6. Enjoy!

Nutritional value

Calories: 278

Carbohydrates: 45g

Cholesterol: 12mg

Fat: 6g

Fiber: 5g

Potassium: 266mg

Protein: 10g

Sodium: 60mg

Sugar: 15g

Mushrooms

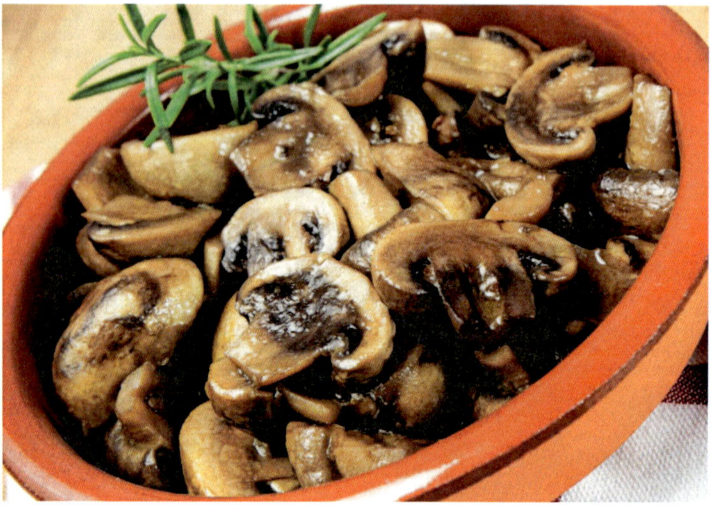

Serving size: 2

Estimated time: 15 minutes

Ingredients

- ¼ kg mushrooms
- 1 cup of baby kale
- 1 tbsp olive oil
- ½ diced onion
- ¼ tbsp black pepper powder
- ¼ tbsp Spanish paprika
- Salt and pepper to taste

Instructions

1. In a pan, heat olive oil under medium heat and fry the onions until they turn golden brown.
2. Add any spices of your choice and stir gently for around 2 minutes.
3. Add kale and cook for 1 minute. They should turn soft at this point.
4. Add salt and pepper and stir to ensure they are well-mixed.
5. Add mushrooms and Sauté for 5 minutes. You can Sauté longer if you wish, depending on the consistency that you desire.
6. Serve and enjoy!
7. Note that you can add avocado if you desire.

Nutritional value per serving

Total fat: 8.2g

Saturated fat: 2.0g

Cholesterol: 164 mg

Total carbs: 6.7g

Protein: 6.8g

Fiber: 6.8g

Sugars: 2g

Vitamin A and C

Iron: 4mg

Niacin: 2mg

Magnesium: 22mg

Folate: 40 mcg

Green Breakfast Smoothie

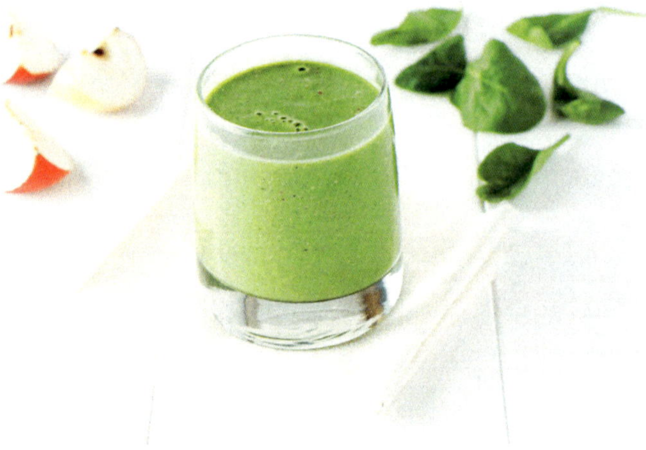

Serving size: 1

Estimated time: 5 minutes

Ingredients

- 1 medium banana
- 1 apple (according to preference)
- 1 cup chopped pineapple
- ⅓ cup fresh Spinach
- 16 oz coconut water
- 1 tbsp. chia seeds

Instructions

1. Prep blender and ingredients.
2. Chop 1 large banana into ¼ length pieces. Add to blender.
3. Quarter the apple. Add to blender.
4. Add pre-chopped pineapple.
5. Add 16 oz coconut water.
6. Add 2 handfuls of fresh spinach.
7. Add chia seeds, if desired.
8. Blend until smooth and serve.

Nutritional Value per Serving

Calories: 473

Lunch / Dinner

Greek Baked Beans

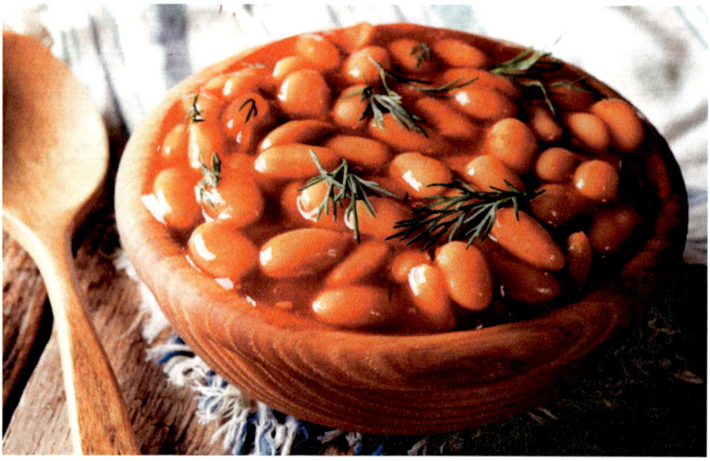

Serving size: 4

Estimated time: 40 minutes

Ingredients

- 1 large onion (finely chopped)
- 1 tbsp tomato purée
- 1 tbsp extra virgin olive oil
- 3 cloves garlic (finely chopped)
- 2 tins chopped tomatoes

- 1 pinch dried oregano/cinnamon
- 1 jar (660g) butter beans (drained and rinsed)
- 2 tbsp chopped parsley
- 4 slices sourdough

Instructions

1. Heat oven and set to 180 degrees.
2. In a large ovenproof frying pan, heat oil, and gently cook onion and garlic. Ensure that you add a pinch of salt to taste.
3. Add tomato purée and cook for at least 1 minute. Add in any spices that you may have (oregano and cinnamon), then add the jar of beans.
4. Add 250 ml of water and bring to a simmer. Remove from heat and put in the oven for 25-30 minutes. At this point, it should have thickened and should be bubbling.
5. Your meal is ready, and you can garnish with chopped parsley. Serve with toasted sourdough or avocado slices.

Nutritional Value per Serving

Calories: 276

Fat: 10g

Sugars (which saturates) 4.8g

Sugars: 11.7g

Fiber: 10.5g

Protein: 15g

Salt: 0.8g

Stir-Fried Tofu Noodles

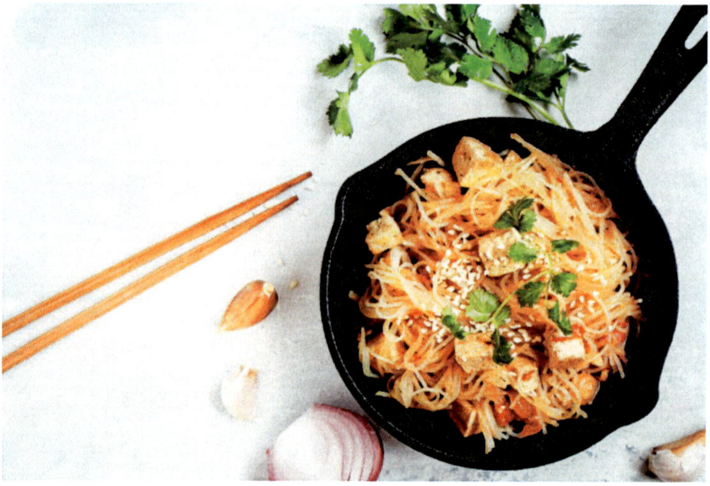

Serving size: 4

Estimated cooking time: 25 minutes

Ingredients

- 225g smoked tofu in cubes
- 2 tbsp sesame oil
- 100g broccoli (cut into chunky pieces)
- 1 carrot (thinly sliced)
- 1 tbsp cornflour
- 2 cloves garlic (crushed)
- 1 tbsp sriracha
- 300g cooked noodles
- 2 spring onions (thinly sliced)

Instructions

1. Place a non-stick pan over high heat and add 2 tbsp sesame oil and some seasoning. Toss tofu for at least 3-4 minutes. You should turn and toss it regularly until it becomes golden all over. Then, tip it out on a kitchen parchment paper.
2. Using sesame oil that remains in the pan, add broccoli, carrots, and bok choy. Stir regularly until it becomes charred at the edges.
3. Take a small bowl and mix together cornflour, soy sauce, and around 100 ml of water. This will make a thick sauce, and you should stir in the garlic and sriracha.
4. Reduce the heat to medium. Then, stir in the sauce.
5. Add in the noodles and mix lightly until everything is well-mixed. Warm gradually until the soup thickens. Your meal is now ready, and you can remove from fire.

6. Serve the noodles with tofu, and top with a sprinkling of spring onions.

Nutritional Value per Serving

Calories: 275

Fat: 7.5g

Fiber: 5.5g

Salt: 1.6g

Protein: 14.2g

Carbohydrates: 35.1g

Saturates: 1.2g

Spinach Muenster Quiche

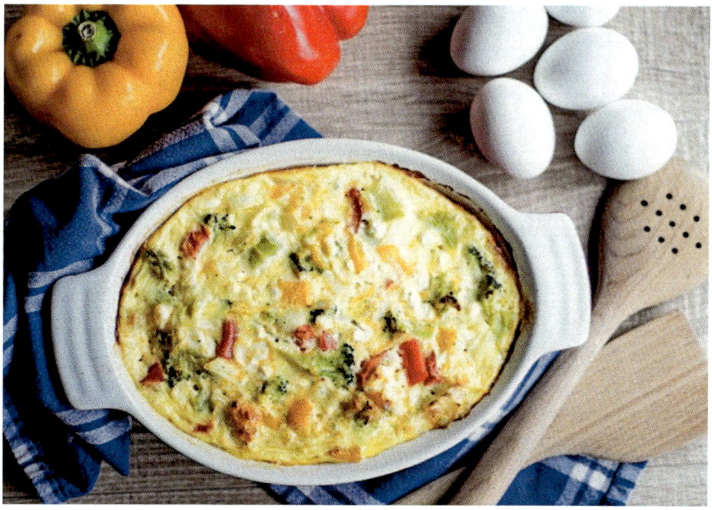

Serving size: 3

Estimated Time: 45 min

Ingredients

- 2 eggs
- 1/3 cup grated cheese (parmesan)
- 8 ounces Muenster cheese (sliced)
- 8-ounce cream cheese (softened)
- Salt and pepper to taste
- 1 pinch garlic powder
- 4 ounces spinach

Instructions

1. Preheat the oven to 350 degrees
2. Line a 9-inch pie pan with 8 ounces Muenster cheese slices
3. Press all water out of spinach and place in a large bowl. Add eggs, parmesan cheese, cream cheese, salt, pepper, and garlic powder. Stir well and gently.
4. Spoon the mixture into the pan and top with the remaining cheese
5. Bake in the oven for 35 minutes. Allow it to set up for 10 minutes then serve.

Nutritional value

Calories: 311

Fat: 25.4g

Carbohydrates: 4.5g

Proteins: 17.8g

Cholesterol: 112mg

Sodium: 484mg

Air Fryer Buffalo Cauliflower

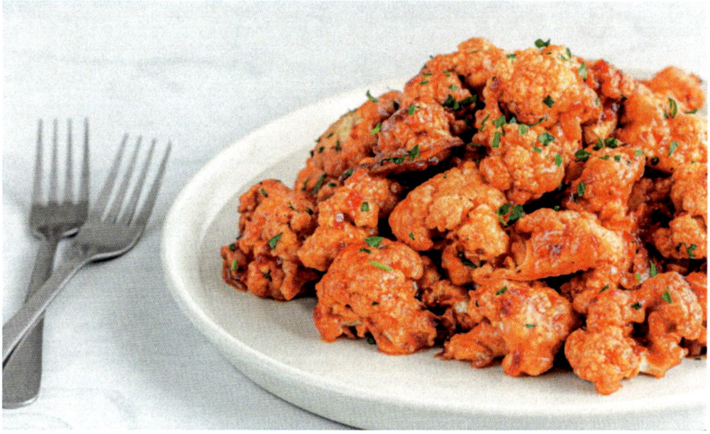

Serving size: 4

Estimated time: 20 minutes

Ingredients

- 4 cups cauliflower florets
- 1 cup panko breadcrumbs. Mix with 1 tbsp. sea salt
- ¼ cup vegan butter (melted)
- ¼ cup buffalo sauce
- Vegan mayonnaise

Instructions

1. Melt the vegan butter in a mug in the microwave. Whisk in the buffalo sauce.

2. Holding the stem, dip each floret in butter/buffalo sauce mixture. Ensure that the entire floret is coated.
3. If the stem does not get saucy, it is okay. Hold up the stem over the mug until it stops dripping.
4. Dredge the florets in the panko/salt mixture and coat as much as you would like. Place in the air fryer.
5. Air fry at 350 degrees F. Note that you should not preheat.
6. Fry for 14-17 minutes and shake gently a few times. When the florets become a little bit browned, you can be sure that it is done.
7. Serve with your preferred dipping sauce.

Nutritional Value

Calories: 22 kcal

Vegetarian Black Bean Enchilada Casserole

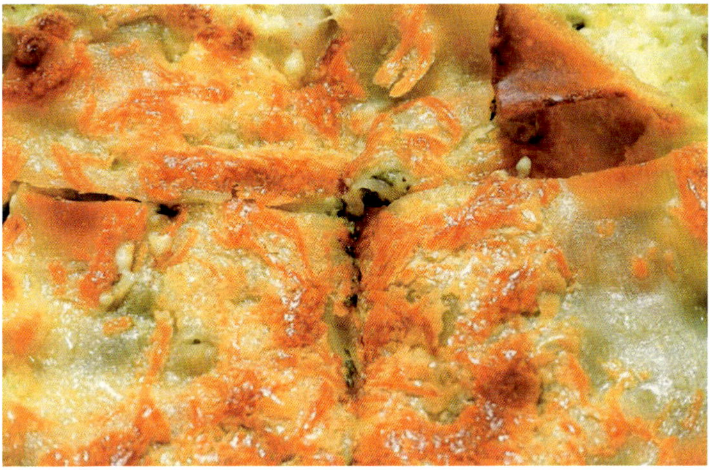

Serving size: 4

Estimated time: 60 minutes

Ingredients

- 28 corn tortillas
- 3 ½ cups enchilada sauce
- 1 red bell pepper (diced)
- 1 tbsp. *el pato* or your favorite jalapeno sauce
- 1 green pepper (diced)
- 1 ½ cups cooked sweet yellow corn kernels
- 2 cans black beans (rinsed and drained)
- Diced cilantro to garnish
- Thinly sliced green onion to garnish

Instructions

1. Preheat the oven to 375 degrees.
2. Grease a 9*13 casserole dish and set aside.
3. Combine enchilada sauce and *el pato* in a sauce until they are fully mixed.
4. Lay 8 tortillas at the bottom of the pan. They can overlap each other
5. Spread 1 ½ cup mixed sauce on the tortillas and ensure that you fully coat them.
6. Sprinkle half the beans, corn, and bell peppers on top of sautéed tortillas. Top with a third of cheese blend.
7. Repeat the layering process. Start with the tortillas, then sauce, then beans, peppers, and cheese.
8. Do this until all the tortillas are used up. Coat the uppermost tortilla with the remaining sauce and sprinkle the cheese on top.
9. Place the pan in the middle rack for 45-55 minutes. Watch the sauce and when it begins bubbling, the enchilada is almost done. At this point, the cheese should have melted and the middle will have cooked through.
10. Remove from oven and leave to cook for 5 minutes.
11. Sprinkle with fresh cilantro and green onions to garnish.
12. Enjoy!

FREE DOWNLOAD

Ultimate Plant-Based Diet Shopping List for Busy People - http://www.plantbasedlyfe.co/

FINAL WORDS

A plant-based diet is one of the best choices that a person can make. The diet has high nutritional value and can solve the worldwide health epidemic. Obesity, cardiovascular issues, diabetes, and related ailments are all largely caused by diet. Luckily, most people have taken life into their own hands. It is for this reason that a plant-based diet continues to grow in popularity. As more realize the benefits, people will live a healthier and more fulfilled life!

Personal Action Plan

An action plan is a short-term roadmap to achieving a goal. People make these to improve their odds of success. Jump-start your plant-based diet journey by filling out your personal action plan.

Step 1. Answer the following questions:

- What do I want to do?
- How much of it do I want to do?
- When (time of day) do I want to do it?
- How often (days of the week) do I want to do it?

Consider the answers to these questions carefully. Remember, switching to a new diet will be a challenge. Remember that "slow and steady" wins the race.

Use this example plan as a reference. *"This week I will ____"*

- What do I want to do? *Eat a plant-based (beef replacement) meal.*
- How much do I want to do? *Start with 1 meal a day.*
- When do I want to do it? *Lunch: 12 p.m.*
- How often do I want to do it? *3 days a week (Monday, Wednesday, Friday)*

Step 2. Determine how confident you are:

Rate yourself on a scale of 1 (not confident) to 10 (fully confident): ______

Note: You should be at a 7 or higher. If not, make sure your plan is realistic.

Step 3: Be accountable

Ask a friend or family member to help you be accountable to your plan. Every week

re-evaluate your plan, and do not quit. When you want to give up, repeat this:

"Nothing tastes as good as healthy feels". Take care and enjoy the journey!

ACKNOWLEDGMENTS

Image Credit: Shutterstock.com